To Marcie

You deserve to live in perfect health!

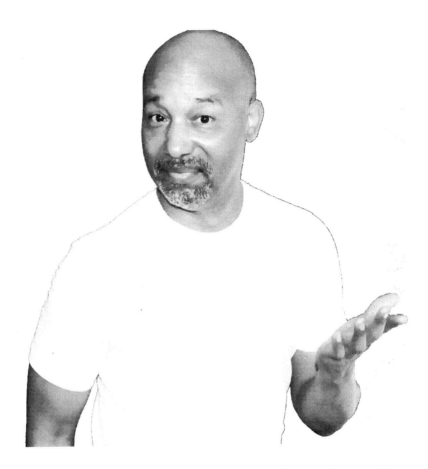

Celebrity chef, a dynamic main-stage speaker, and one of the most productive health-research writers for the generation, **Chef Keidi Awadu** is on a powerful mission to spread his unique gospel of perfect health. Audiences are consistently amazed at a depth of health-science wisdom that Chef Keidi serves up to support his claim that "Food is Nature's most perfect medicine and medicine has *never* tasted like this before." He is the creator of the **Living Superfood** brand of nutrition-dense, raw vegan cuisine, as well as the author of six books touting the Living Superfood clinical nutrition system.

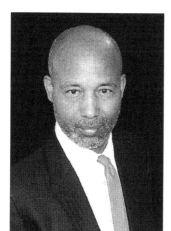

FROM THE LIVING SUPERFOOD SERIES

GET THE WEIGHT OFF
– 30-Days to a New You

Created and compiled by Keidi Awadu,
aka The Conscious Rasta
Copyright 2012 by Keidi Awadu
Revised March 2018
Published by the Conscious Rasta Press
9515 W. Cherrydale Ct.,
Las Vegas NV 89147 U.S.A.
All rights reserved under U.S. copyright law

Library of Congress Cataloging-in-Publication Data is available from the publisher. This book, or parts thereof, may not be reproduced in any form without permission from the publisher; with exceptions made for brief excerpts used in published reviews.

This publication is designed to provide accurate and authoritative information about the subject matter covered. It is distributed with the understanding that the publisher and author are not engaged in rendering legal, accounting, medical or other professional advice. If such advice is required, the services of a competent professional person should be engaged whenever possible. Decisions made regarding the health of the reader are the sole responsibility of the reader and not the author and publisher of this book.

The above photo is courtesy of Choice Imagery, Baltimore / ChoiceImagery.com

We have a wonderful set of DVD's to compliment this book at **LivingSuperFood.com**. You can follow Chef Keidi at **ChefKeidi.com**.

E-mail me (Keidi@chefkeidi.com) for those who want to have a workshop, catering, personal consultation or other interaction on this wonderful new way of living and eating. The telephone number to reach me directly is 323.902.2919.

GET THE WEIGHT OFF – 30 Days to a New You

Introduction – The New Life Paradigm 1

Chapter 1 – Set and Get Your Goals 3

Who? What? When? Where?.. 3

Obesity Causes & Consequences 3

Get a digital scale and weigh yourself every day. 6

Drink more water 6

Today and every day eat raw fruits and vegetables. 7

Begin Each Day with 15-20 Minutes of Exercise 8

Journaling as a way of affirming the journey....................... 9

Bring a friend along on your journey. 10

Chapter 2 – Let's Think this Through 13

Getting Friends and Family Involved.................................. 13

Dealing with Unwarranted Fears and Anxiety 14

Nutritional Supplementation 15

Being a Mature Person in a Young Person's Body 16

Sharing and Showing Off our Healthy Gourmet Cuisine..... 18

Beyond the Grip of a New Enslavement 19

Mass Media Promotes Malnutrition Across the Society 21

Chapter 3 – If It's About Money, Consider This 23

America's Skyrocketing Cost of Healthcare 23

The Government Is NOT the Solution 24

Overweight and Obesity and the Cost of Healthcare 25

Being Sick is a Waste of Labor Potential 26

A Vegan Lifestyle Inserts More Time in Your Day 26

How to Spot Fake Food When You Go Shopping................. 28

Stop Wasting Money on Depleted Food 31

Chapter 4 – Childhood and Teen Obesity 33

Seeds Sown for Future Crises 33

Shocking Facts about Child and Teen Obesity 33

Are Your Children What *You* Eat? 36

The Family Meal – Is S.A.D. the Best You Can Do? 36

The Sedentary Child in American Society 37

Changing Household Habits 38

Keeping Our Youth Enthusiastic About Life 38

Chapter 5 – A Radical New Concept of "Dieting" 41

Why I Don't Advocate Dieting 41

Counting Calories is Pointless and Distracting 42

The Digestive System is Smarter Than You Think 44

How the Body Switches to High-Efficiency 46

Lose Weight" While Eating Growth Hormones? 47

Full-Spectrum Hyper Nutrition to the Rescue 48

Burn Body Fat Without Starving 51

Chapter 6 – Women's Weight and "The Burden" 54

What Do the Numbers Say? 54

Reversing Obesity-Related Disease 57

More Time in Your Days; More Days in Your Life 61

Chapter 7 – Four Stages of Healing 64

Stage 1 – Removing the Underlying Cause of Disease 65

Stage 2 – Relief From Symptoms 69

Stage 3 – Feeling the Energy Within 71

Stage 4 – Rejuvenation 74

The 7 Principles of Optimal Health 75

Introduction – The New Life Paradigm

I have set upon the task of stretching the boundaries of your imagination and beliefs throughout this edition of the **New Conscious Rasta Report**™. While much of what follows explores levels of biological sciences such as nutrition, human anatomy, molecular biology and medical science, for the most part, I intend on keeping to relatively simple concepts and easy-to-follow logic. The imagination is a wonderfully fertile space in which limitless possibilities can be presented and understood.

Key concepts such as natural, environment, disorder, rejuvenation, holistic and psycho-spirituality will bear repetition throughout the book. The journey which we are representing herein begins within the mind, through practical concepts and principles of health. The logical and intended end of this commitment will be a refreshed outlook on Life and a brand new physiological standard for your body.

When we come to think of ourselves and what we deserve in life, most of us regard ourselves as good and worthy people. We would like to believe that we are honest, hardworking, deserving and grateful. Yet, the reality of how we present ourselves to the larger community is all too often in direct conflict with such noble values. I have become convinced that to go through decades of our life in stages of chaos, disorder, disease and depression is a major conflict between perceptions of self, what we deserve and that which is so often settled for.

If you are settling for the symptoms of premature aging, fatigue, lacking a feeling of well-being, or somehow thinking that you are ashamed of yourself in some manner, then you may want to consider that it's time for a "**New Life Paradigm.**" You just may be due to being "born again" in some fashion of mind, body, and spirit – or all of these. This report *GET THE WEIGHT OFF – 30 Days to a New You* is written with the specific intention to correct issues within the body which have created a chaotic state upon which disorder produces disease, which is evident with specific symptoms.

There is undeniably an epidemic of overweight and obesity occurring around the world, and this is especially evident in the richer, developed nations. Certain ethnic classes are experiencing this crisis worse than others, and it is also affecting women at a higher rate than men. The crisis has gone on so long without a logical resolution to the point that it has now reached firmly into the youth population. Thus, this crisis of overweight and obesity promises to worsen over the course of generations unless there is a widespread paradigm shift.

The **New Life Paradigm** will present itself as a miracle to some and as a logical outcome to others. Either way, it is necessary as it is evident that we cannot continue along the same path of unconscious eating and disease causation.

So give us your attention, imagination, focus, and commitment over the course of the next thirty days. There is a miracle that has just been waiting for you to claim it.

Chapter 1 – Set and Get Your Goals

Who? What? When? Where?

"Who am I? What do I want to accomplish? Where am I headed in life and when do I *plan* on arriving at my destination?"

Like everything else in life, "those who fail to plan, plan to fail." The same is true with our bodies. We need to have a strong vision of ourselves as healthy, prosperous, energetic and youthful. That image of self must become pervasive, accompany us every hour of every day and we need not be hypocrites about carrying such an image. Still, this state of eternal youthfulness need NOT be dependent upon hair dyes (toxic), makeup (toxic), dieting (starvation) or medical procedures (stupid and unnecessary). Deal with the fact of your overweight status by 1) acknowledging that you got out of control over time, 2) making a realistic goal of where you intend to be, and 3) picking a reasonable date upon which you will have declared your *first* victory.

Obesity Causes & Consequences

Let's get this painful revelation out of the way early in the book. Overweight and obesity represent a spectrum of problems. These present social problems, health, longevity, personal convenience, and logistic problems. Our perception of body image and anxiety over how others think about us profoundly impacts our mental health.

Being overweight should be no measure of a person's character, worth or values as a human being. Overweight people are lively, loyal, creative, funny, disciplined and lovable. Overweight people are just like you and me as complete human beings. Too often, overweight people are distracted by their physical presence to the point that it interferes with the spectrum of affairs which should better occupy their attention. Overweight people, like everyone else in this world, need a little more love, empathy, and respect in their daily lives.

Obesity is another level of challenge because it can be associated with increased risk of a spectrum of disorders and diseases. Overweight becomes obesity when these medical issues appear and become increasingly problematic. Overweight is unpleasant and inconvenient. Obesity is dangerous because it directly associates with morbidity and mortality—disease and death.

There is a terrible burden of obesity-related diseases and disorders that are plaguing the world's population today. The following is perhaps the most comprehensive list you will have ever seen of these obesity-related diseases and disorders.

1. All causes of death are affected by overweight and obesity

2. Cardiovascular diseases such as atherosclerosis (plaque buildup in the arteries), a precursor to many other disorders

3. Increased heart rate

4. Coronary heart disease

5. Stroke (cerebral embolism)

6. Pulmonary embolism

7. Angina (chest pain)

8. Cancers of the endometrium, breast, colon, kidney, gallbladder, uterus, prostate, and liver

9. Type 2 diabetes and insulin resistance

10. Metabolic syndrome

11. Gallbladder disease

12. Fatty liver disease

13. Kidney disease (chronic nephropathy)

14. Gout (excessive uric acid in the blood)

15. Systemic inflammation

16. Asthma

17. Musculoskeletal disorders (bone diseases)

18. Osteoarthritis (breakdown of cartilage and bone in joints)

19. Hip and knee replacement surgery

20. Sleep apnea and breathing difficulties

21. Hypertension (high blood pressure)

22. High LDL cholesterol

23. Dyslipidemia (elevated levels of triglycerides)

24. Gestational diabetes during pregnancy and risk of C-section delivery

25. Psychological effects such as depression and mental disorders

26. Social stigmatizing and reduced quality of life

27. Systemic body pain and poor physical functioning

28. Generalized malnutrition

29. Risks associated with gastric surgery

30. Diet drug addiction

31. Yeast infection

This spectrum of obesity-associated disorders is shocking. This realization is overwhelming. You have made a firm decision that you do not want to live (and die) like this. Let's get to work on creating a new paradigm within which you have taken control.

Get a digital scale and weigh yourself every day.

I weighed in today (March 2018) at 154 lbs. This weight is perfectly within the range of my optimal physical condition. Every day I look forward to getting on the scale. I do so in the morning just after my bowel movement and before I start the day with two 12-ounce glasses of purified water. Many people who are overweight avoid the scale because they don't like the disappointing news it has most often been reporting. I advise getting on the scale for just the opposite reason – because you love the *good news* that it reports about your ongoing transformation. Start TODAY and don't put this off for another moment. Within 2 to 7 days your scale will be the first to congratulate you every morning.

Drink more water

Many people don't realize the many ways that dehydration brings disorder to our physical nature. Our bodies are 70%

water, just like Planet Earth. If 10 percent of Earth's surface disappeared, it would bring massive chaos, disorder, and destruction to the species inhabiting it. The same is true for our bodies. Most of the public is dehydrated to some stage most of the time. Only a small percentage of people consume enough water or water-containing natural foods to be considered properly hydrated. Remember that coffee, sodas, energy drinks and high-fructose corn syrup fake fruit juices are in actuality *anti-water* and will cause more dehydration problems than they solve.

Today and every day eat raw fruits and vegetables.

Put some *color* in a big salad bowl, eat lots of fiber-containing foods and stuff your intestinal tract with *energy-producing, vegan superfoods*.

I'll have much to say during our month together about *why* one must avoid acid-forming foods to normalize one's weight. But for now, **here is a group of DON'T EATS you want to avoid** as much as possible (like *completely*) during this 30-Day transformation if your goal is to *GET THE WEIGHT OFF*:

1. Coffee, sodas, energy drinks and high-fructose corn syrup (HFCS) loaded fake juices;

2. Red meat (beef, pork, lamb), poultry (chicken, turkey — they're contaminated with growth hormones, steroids, and antibiotics AND are acid-forming), as well as are eggs;

3. If you feel you must eat seafood (which you don't), avoid scavengers and eat only open-sea cold-water fish like

salmon or cod. Avoid farm-raised fish and ocean-bottom feeders.

4. Avoid pasta (glue-like wheat gluten) and bread (inflammatory and carcinogenic). Raw bread can be tolerated but could also be avoided for 30 days. Substitute leafy greens for bread if you want to enjoy a healthy sandwich.

5. Dairy, including low-fat products, cheese, milk-based yogurt, whey products, anything that contains casein (glue made from milk), to include both cow and goat milk products;

6. There will be more tips on things to avoid or eliminate as our program continues.

Begin Each Day with 15-20 Minutes of Exercise

Not only do we need to find ways of burning all that excess fuel our bodies store, but we need to move to open channels of blood, energy and oxygen flow within the body. Stop thinking of exercise as "burning calories" – that is more of that *dieting crap* that the *mis-informers* rely upon to keep people dependent upon their inefficient programs. Yes, when we move our cells burn fuel, it happens all day long. Better yet, we can get energy flowing throughout the body. Those who practice low-stress exercises like Tai Chi are also able to maintain the proper balance of their weight. It is all about *the flow of energy*, and yours has become bottled up and stored as fat in the wrong places, especially if you sit all day at the job.

9 | Chapter 1 – Set and Get Your Goals

Journaling as a way of affirming the journey

Begin an audio or written journal of this 30-day journey. Use your powerful voice to project your goals and affirmations.

Somewhere in your subconscious mind, you may have disordered your relationship to your body, and to Nature. You have chosen this month to reboot because you felt disconnected from your creativity, discipline, as well as disconnected from important relationships with others.

If you are with the Reboot because you have been engaging in "chewicide," then it is critical that you get rid of that anxiety-ridden invader that is sabotaging your healthy lifestyle. Journaling, both audio and written, along with speaking affirmations, are ways that we can get into our deepest feelings and redirect energy to the empowered Self within.

Affirm your strengths. Affirm your self-worth. Give voice to what you do that is the best of the best ABOVE others who do the same as you do. As my Baba Les Brown frequently reminds us, "You have Greatness within you," and he is *absolutely* correct with this admonition. When you hear his commanding instruction, again and again, you will search deeper within to extract that greatness that you are ordering to surface and project itself to the world.

Let's put a few simple steps on the table for immediate goals to fulfill our thirty-day mission. These are proven to help us move forward rapidly to achieve our desired goals.

1) While a written journal is best, let's be honest and admit that a lot of us feel too busy to write nowadays. Fortunately,

we can access pocket audio recorders or cell phones with easy-to-use recorders built right in. You have spare time throughout the day you can use to affirm your most important goals for the month. Use your cell phone to record these goals or, better yet, write them down as well. Talk to yourself and affirm these goals repeatedly using your powerful voice.

2) Is your plan to get rid of 15 pounds of excess weight? Do you want to stop depending on pharmaceutical drugs? How about an increase in strength, stamina and vital energy? Whatever your goals, reduce them to short and simple language, and embed these phrases in your mind. "I will strengthen my breathing this month through vigorous exercise." "With 400 squat thrusts a day, I will have legs as strong as a man half my age." "I will extend my lifespan by detoxing daily." Clarify your goals, refine and shorten the language. Then affirm them throughout the day using your powerful voice.

3) Speak your affirmations to the world. Share your goals with friends, family, coworkers, and those in your Reboot support circle. Be clear when you give voice to these goals, don't stutter and NEVER sound as if you lack confidence. Now is where that Powerful Voice comes with full authority. In the beginning is the WOOOORD! Speak into existence what you expect of yourself and what the world should expect from you.

Bring a friend along on your journey.

Like all other species, humans do their best work in cooperative partnership. For your 30-day Reboot, bring a friend, your significant other, a parent, child or co-worker along on the journey. It will be much more pleasurable, you will help to

11 | Chapter 1 — Set and Get Your Goals

reinforce each other, and you will have a readily-available buddy-coach to help you set critical goals and stick to them.

Every day that we awaken, we have the chance to forge great new possibilities. Directionless, we can become suckered into lives of *virtual* enslavement. Being unfocused is one of the main causes of resentment about Life that leads to *chewicide* and other self-destructive behaviors. Think about it — We are divine beings, created within the Master's Plan and endowed with all of the possibilities which constitute a great life. Each day that you're alive, you must validate your uniqueness, creativity, self-motivation, and "purpose-fullness."

Repeat after me: "Through the actions that I do today, by living and acting within the 'now-ness' of my existence, I reward myself with tremendous benefits, along with appreciation from those with whom I share the world." [Repeat as much as needed!]

You, I, WE deserve to be healthy, wealthy, wise and appreciated. We validate this deserving condition with our actions. Therefore, we are eager to put in the work. We give generously. We give vision to bold new accomplishments and have every intention of becoming powerful change-agents affecting every aspect of the world of today and tomorrow.

What are a few transforming changes you want to make in the world?

1) Meditate on this question for a minute before you translate it to seven words or less. "Use scientific knowledge to affect profound changes." "Be the best father for my daughters." "Inspire eight billion people to eat healthier." Seven words

can change the world. Take the time to craft your message with precise power. "Next month I'll enjoy tremendously improved health!"

2) Find those around you who share your mission and who you can infect with your enthusiasm. We'd like to help everyone we can, but don't drag deadbeat energy along with you on this trip. Make a list of everyone who you regularly encounter and rank them for their ability to support your dreams, your mission and your unshakable determination to succeed.

3) Take what we are learning this month and move it beyond the boundaries of the Reboot. I can promise you that we are going to cover a lot of valuable ground during our 30-Days to a New You journey. But you're going to have to want it beyond my coaching alone. Again, quoting my Baba Les Brown, "You gotta be Hungry!" Your partners in this journey must support your drive, your passion and your hunger for change. When two of you join on such a mission, it is much more likely that a third, fourth or a dozen more will want to come with you. Find your collaborators and convince them that you will all do best to succeed together in this and everything else to which you commit.

Man, am I *excited* about what we're doing here. Life IS MAGNIFICENT! And we all show great intentionality when it comes to proving this again today and every day, even beyond the 30 days of the Reboot.

Chapter 2 – Let's Think this Through

Getting Friends and Family Involved

I regularly host an amazingly-productive conference call with participants from across the nation and abroad participating. A typical weight-reduction teleconference will typically showcase major points about disease prevention brought up during our 60-minute discussions. We discuss many insightful health issues. I want to share some of these session highlights with you.

Many of us have been preaching to those around us as if healthy living were religion. Think about your reaction when someone you didn't ask attempted to persuade you to *their* religious journey. If you're like me, it wasn't a pleasant or welcome experience. It's probably best to not be so imposing.

Why not just carry healthy food around with you as you move through your world, with enough surpluses that you can offer some to others? Why not just become a shining example of health to the point that others comment and inquire as to your secret? Also, show genuine interest in what others are into, take time to listen to their concerns, visions, inner conflicts, joys, and ambitions.

Chances are, at a certain point people will trust you and thus open more to your ideas. Too often those of us who fixate on health and longevity lose sight that their passions motivate every individual. If we would wish that people share ours then we had probably better convince them that we sincerely want to share their passions and concerns as well – it's called *reciprocity.* Thus, the first part of becoming a more effective change agent is to become a better role model and listener.

Dealing with Unwarranted Fears and Anxiety

At the heart of many people's battles with food and other substance abuse is a torment of anxiety, psychic trauma, and insecurity. Everybody needs *freedom and dignity* to feel positive about their life as it relates to those around them. Unfounded fears and anxieties handicap too many lives. One of the more common anxieties is an unreasonable fear of future criticism; being worried about what people will think or say after some future action *might* occur at some future time. In such cases, that feared castigation has probably been going on in their head and keeps them from challenging habits that impede positive transformation.

WHO CARES about what somebody MIGHT SAY if you make a life change? If people do offer *negative* criticism, reserve the right to only accept it as *positive*, thus allowing oneself the chance to grow from the experience. When we consider all criticism as an opportunity for rapid growth, we then can't help but welcome it.

The society in which most of us find ourselves today is full of deceivers and fools. As profit-driven corporations shove more and more corrupted food down the throats of a vulnerable public, they use their wealth to proliferate ideas that consuming their toxic junk is *normal* and that a life without the common desires of the average consumer is weird.

Thus, the highly intelligent young person is labeled *nerd*. Self-disciplined individuals are called *prudish*. An inquiring mind is

15 | Chapter 2 – Let's Think this Through

labeled a *conspiracy nut*. And the one who shows caution in the manner that they deal with nutrition is branded a health *nut* or dismissed as a social misfit. So be it. In a society of stupid people, it is radical to be pragmatic and intelligent in one's decisions.

Today, Fat America calls slender people bitter names (likely reversing torment that slender people so often put on their heavier compatriots a generation earlier). There are those who think that slim people are weak, anemic, impotent and psychologically damaged. How many times can people laugh at a comedienne who condemns slender and youthful women by cursing them as "skinny b**ch's?" Who was the joke really on when you one day find yourself clutching your chest and struggling to survive a heart attack?

Don't allow the Big Lie to steal away your common sense. Slender people are strong, health-abundant, purposeful and sexually-charged. The myth is busted.

Nutritional Supplementation

While it would be wrong for me to deny a range of benefits one can acquire by supplementing, my experience shows that once I moved into a whole food, plant-based vegan, and raw food lifestyle, I was using supplements less and less. These days I mostly only supplement when I am fasting – when I am deliberately *starving* my body as part of a seasonal cleanse, or if I have some reason to counter some manner of stresses in my routine. At those times, when I may be consuming only water or prune juice for a period of up to 5-10 days, vitamin, mineral and herbal supplements are critically needed. These supplements most often make a substantial difference toward tolerance of a fast.

For most of the season, I am eating a broad spectrum of fruits, vegetables, roots, nuts, seeds, grains, oils, culinary herbs, etc. and my nutritional pattern is so broad that I don't feel much need to take additional supplements. Therefore, supplements are good, but you should not have to rely on them all of the time for extending your nutrition. Exceptions might be when 1) you perceive you are experiencing disorder related to nutrient deficiency; 2) you are engaging in detoxification fast, or 3) you suspect that much of the foods you are eating is grown in nutrient-deficient soil.

Being a Mature Person in a Young Person's Body

It sound's kinda lecherous and nasty when we're thinking about an older person wanting to "get inside" a young person's body. Sexually, true – that is usually a way of out-of-bounds. But today I want to engage your imagination to an earlier time of your *own* physical self.

Take your current age and divide it in half; how old were you then? At that age how did you feel about your body? How much did you weigh when you were between the ages of 21 and 28 at the peak of your adult hormonal integrity? Did you feel strong, energetic, and excited about life? Did you feel invincible?

Adult's glandular integrity begins to degrade in their late thirties. Body parts begin to show some wear and tear. It might be a shift in our eyesight; we may run out of breath sooner when exercising or playing sports. People start to gain

17 | Chapter 2 — Let's Think this Through

anywhere from 1 to 5 pounds each year from that point of their lives, and the muscle weight we used to carry high in the torso starts to shift downward, toward the mid-section.

The fact is, for most people natural aging processes start to advance and become more noticeable as the decades pass. This natural process is called "senescence," and it happens to everyone on the organic, cellular and genetic levels.

But WHAT IF you could learn to slow down, arrest or even reverse this aging process? What if the strategies that you willfully put into place allowed you to take advantages of food and nutrition as a reliable "fountain of youth?"

When a mature man or woman transforms their body with full-spectrum hyper-nutrition, breath management, hydration, exercise, detoxification, rest and a bright outlook on life, they rejuvenate to the point that they transform themselves into restored youthfulness.

Better yet, one retains one's mature experiences, insights, accumulated wisdom, discipline and acquired values. It is as if you get to live the second half of your chronological years all over again, only this time you are beneficiary of your chronologically-accumulated wisdom.

There's another bonus to being able to live the second half of your years again. This time you can regulate aging at a much slower pace with the same practices that contributed to rejuvenation. This breakthrough understanding is why some of us are staking the claim to expected lifespans of as much as 120 years in this generation.

Here are three simple instructions you can quickly and conveniently incorporate into your regime.

1) Take an assessment of your present physical status and compare it to that of yourself at half your current age.

2) Take the rest of this 30-day course and build up to an exercise routine that begins to move you toward your earlier performance. If you are like me, you can achieve twice the rate of strength that you demonstrated at half your current age.

3) Take advantage of youthfulness coaching and build up a library centered around longevity, restoring and retaining your youthfulness, as well as study how to maintain optimal functioning within the body's systems without resorting to artificial means.

What a joy it is to be half one's current years again. It is simply AMAZING! •

Sharing and Showing Off our Healthy Gourmet Cuisine

For years I was a competent vegan chef and took immense pride in sharing my craft with others. Now that I have advanced to the level that I *know* beyond a doubt that **Living Superfood**™ cuisine is a healing art as well, my pride in showcasing this food has ever increased. When you master this cuisine, after months of living it and exploring your culinary heights, you can speak with absolute confidence to those who might be reluctant to try it out. Not everybody is going to enjoy it, and some will not even want to give it a taste; that's okay. You know in your own heart what this is about and as such you can feel confident that

19 | Chapter 2 – Let's Think this Through

no matter what others think, your self-worth is intact. No worry...there's more for me to eat.

Beyond the Grip of a New Enslavement

History teaches of the notorious *Triangular Trade* through which European enslavers kidnapped and shipped human chattel from the west coast of Africa into the Americas. Upon arrival, these enslaved were forced into brutal labor, producing sugar, rum, and cotton for export to Europe. Upon arrival, these commodities derived from slavery generated huge profits for those who financed this unholy era of mercantilism, further targeting innocent Africans for another round of mass kidnapping.

Paradoxically, since the time of outlawing slavery, a new and equally sinister Triad has risen, consisting of the following:

1) Processed food manufacturers, junk food, and fast food distributors peddle toxic products which cause widespread pathology among those who are their most loyal consumers;

2) Sickened by malnutrition, the affected population seeks relief from the healthcare providers, who are making windfall profits marketing ineffective medical procedures and equally toxic (and sickening) drugs toward the aim of suppressing the symptoms caused by food-associated pathologies;

3) Government regulatory agencies (FDA, USDA, DHHS, NCI, CDC, FTC, etc.) which are *supposed* to be protecting the population through regulation of these corporations, turn a blind eye to the massive injury caused by consuming these

toxic products. Aspirant underlings to corporate bosses getting paid fat wages to head the exploitive medical cartels, frequently manage these so-called "consumer protection agencies."

This premise of a new Triangular Trade is provocative, yet I am speaking to a truth which I know very well. A big difference between this new holocaust and that of past centuries is that today *our participation as the enslaved is overwhelmingly a voluntary process*. From early in life, various societal influences direct us to choices that entangle us in this deadly exploitation.

Our purpose during the 30-Day Reboot is to choose to exit the field upon which this deadly game continually plays out. We simply must stop consuming foods that we *know* make us ill, a process I've termed "chewicide." We can, and we must move with deliberation toward conscious eating of the most appropriate nutrition and engage in other practices like regular detoxification. This simple yet effective solution will go a long way to create space in our lives for perfect health.

Here are three more simple calls to action to stay beyond the reach of this new enslavement:

1) Realize the consequences of how your dietary habits have an impact on your long-term health. Old habits die hard, yet new habits are quick to start. Create habitual patterns that compliment your intention to improve your nutritional lifestyle.

2) We must take our charge seriously to use other alternatives to pharmaceutical drugs to suppress symptoms. Because you accept the premise that Food is Nature's Most Perfect

21 | Chapter 2 – Let's Think this Through

Medicine, you are now able to craft solutions to disorders and diseases which rely upon food-based strategies for healing.

3) Come to terms that a spectrum of government agencies are failing to protect the public from an assault by junk food industries, injury from ineffective medical practices, and that vast segment of the business community which consistently puts profits before people.

You will have to take primary responsibility for these critical decisions. You are not alone. Many other effective coaches and I will be available to assist you to make dramatic habitual shifts. The battle against chewicide is being won every day in every community. You are not alone. You just may have underestimated the tactical organization of those who have been exploiting our nutritional vulnerability.

Just as the world has proclaimed that we will never again subject humans to the holocaust of forced enslavement, we pledge to refuse to cooperate with this new enslavement of unhealthy food, even worse medicine, and terrible protection from government agencies.

Mass Media Promotes Malnutrition Across the Society

This culture of mass consumption has taken a century to develop to the point that many big lies have become pervasive throughout society. Newspapers, magazines, radio, television, movies and now the Internet all are utilized as vehicles of mass deception. We're being told by mass media what is proper to wear, what to drink, eat, smoke, paint on our bodies, put in our bloodstream and how to celebrate the fundamental traditions of life. Most people aren't particularly conscious of what they accept as legitimate via mass media.

Television has become "Tell-Lie-Vision," and we now have about four generations growing up tethered to this *mischievous electronic umbilical cord.* We need to elevate the standard of media literacy and train the population, especially youth, to resist being conned into accepting that which is unnatural and corrupting. For many households, it could be as simple as unplug the cable and only allow media to serve as a platform for academic assistance. Repurposing these media is not going to be an easy task...but it sure is rewarding!

As you can see, we are going to have a magnificent journey for these 30 days. Won't you consider joining us? Go to the web site **LivingSuperFood.com** and get on board. You don't want to miss THIS train. Get on board before it leaves the station.

Chapter 3 - If It's About Money, Consider This

America's Skyrocketing Cost of Healthcare

Many people believe that healthy nutrition, and many routines that contribute to it, are prohibitive because of the expenses involved. I believe the opposite—that it is cheaper to be healthy. I will share several insights to demonstrate this efficiency of health. As well I'll share tips as to how I maintain optimal health on a very reasonable budget.

I often talk about the savings that you could expect when you apply the 7 Principles of Optimal Health (breath, water, food, exercise, rest, detoxification and mind state). In recent years I have used the figure of $10,000 spent on average per person on healthcare in the U.S. annually. The following news article uses a figure of $8233-per-person (combined public and private expenses) for 2010. (from the *NY Times, June 28, 2012*: **U.S. HEALTH COSTS MORE THAN 'SOCIALIZED' EUROPEAN MEDICINE**, by Harvey Morris)

> Combined public and private spending on health care in the U.S. came to $8,233 per person in 2010, more than twice as much as relatively rich European countries such as France, Sweden and Britain that provide universal health care.
>
> Are Americans healthier as a result? The U.S. has fewer doctors per capita than comparable countries and fewer hospital beds. But more is spent on advanced diagnostic equipment and health tests.

Life expectancy has risen in line with that in other developed countries, but the average American life span of 78.7 years in 2010 was below the O.E.C.D. average. Obesity in the U.S. was the highest in the 34-nation survey.

If we add an additional 6% annual increase in U.S. healthcare expenses for the years that have followed, then by 2018 that per capita healthcare expense will exceed $13,000 yearly. The bottom line is that with proper management of our body's natural tendency toward maintaining health with the right environment, we can cut this annual expense in half for most people. What is needed is preventative medicine, also referred to as *functional medicine*. We thus have, on average, over $252 a week expended on what is sadly called "healthcare" in the U.S. Investing just half of that, $126 per week, in healthy lifestyle maintenance would be a great investment toward transforming our health.

The Government Is NOT the Solution

A few years back I produced a documentary film, *Chewicide*. In the film, I showed how a combination of:

1) The proliferation of toxic among the American population had produced an outcome of widespread disease and disorder;

2) This disorder led to disproportionate consumption of pharmaceutical drugs and medical procedures for which a medical-industrial complex was making a gross profit from the public's poor health status; and

3) That food industries and healthcare industries were dedicating a portion of their gross receipts to lobby legislatures

25 | Chapter 3 — If It's About Money, Consider This

and regulatory agencies to allow them to continue exploiting this system without fear of significant blowback.

What I was describing was a new form of enslavement — a new *Triangular Slave Trade*. I suggested that it was an exact parallel to the Triangular Trade that developed the unholy history of chattel slavery in the Western hemisphere.

The unwelcome conclusion is, for the foreseeable future and multiple reasons, we will not be able to rely upon government agencies to correct the vast problems within the nation's healthcare system. How many of us would thus feel that our optimal health is so important that we are compelled to arrange to make needed changes apart from the intent of public and private interests? My **Living Superfood** program is a fantastic way to take back your share of the $3.9 trillion annual investment in being only marginally healthy in America.

Overweight and Obesity and the Cost of Healthcare

According to a Reuters article from April 30, 2012, excess expenses in America due to this nation's high rate of overweight and obesity is estimated at $190 billion annually; nearly 1/5th of the national healthcare expense. The expenses can be classified several ways:

- Lost productivity (obese men take an average of six more sick days a year while obese women use nine more sick days over their non-obese coworkers per year)

- I have identified a host of 31 medical conditions associated with obesity, ranging from cardiovascular disease and hypertension to chronic pain, cancer and a spectrum of digestive issues. Pediatric obesity is another area of rapidly increasing medical expenses.

- "Obese men rack up an additional $1,152 per year in medical spending, especially hospitalizations and prescription drugs... Obese women account for an extra $3,613 a year." Among the uninsured, "annual medical spending for an obese person was $3,271 compared with $512 for the non-obese."

Being Sick is a Waste of Labor Potential

Not only are many work days lost to the consequences of weight-related disabilities, but our desire and capacity to engage in physical activity are severely limited. It's hard to get and stay motivated when we are tired from hauling around a mass of stored energy with us all day long. Constant craving for food can distract one from concentrating on critical tasks at hand. Our work should be a joy, a true labor of love. While there is no cause to believe that overweight people are not passionate and committed to productive work, still we would give ourselves every advantage to be able to be highly efficient workers. Being in great shape is a compliment to any venture upon which we would engage.

A Vegan Lifestyle Inserts More Time in Your Day

Many people report what I have experienced since going 98% raw over the past 2 ½ years. Raw vegans have reduced the need for sleep by about two hours a day. Also, that feeling of drowsiness referred to as *"The Itis"* which one gets after eating a large meal, rarely occurs when one isn't experiencing

27 | C h a p t e r 3 — I f I t's A b o u t M o n e y, C o n s i d e r T h i s

digestive leukocytosis because of eating dead food. Thus, you can recover 2 more hours a day, 14 hours a week, *over 30 days a year* by just eating smarter.

As well, shopping smart saves money. I have developed various techniques for saving at the grocery stores and markets I frequent. I hope some of the following shopping strategies work for you:

- Farmers markets have a broad selection of fresh produce, often organic, and you can sometimes get even better deals buying by the case or shopping near the close of the market for the day. Harsh weather days save the most if the market is open as these marketers certainly don't want to have to reload all of their aging produce to chance on another opportunity to sell it while it is still fresh.

- Neighborhood stores will often have one day a week where fresh produce is on sale. Yesterday I carried seven bags of fruits and vegetables home for under $15 from my regular Wednesday stop.

- Shopping online for certain items can bring substantial savings on items like nuts, seeds, dried fruits and specialty products, even when shipping expenses figure into the price.

- Buy those items you will use a lot in larger packaging. That can cut out a sizable percentage of the cost-per-serving.

- Ask the store manager if you can have that case of bananas, apples or tomatoes that they are pulling off the stand. Stores often throw away food that is perfect for our juicing, dehydrating or food processing needs. I have frequently bought whole cases of bananas for a mere $3 or $4, as well as other produce. Just because it's bruised or spotted doesn't mean that it is unfit for consumption. Stores throw away a lot of food.

- Stop allowing produce to rot in your refrigerator. Clean shelves and bottom drawers of your fridge a couple of times a week and stop having to throw away spoiled food.

- Do-It-Yourself (DIY) and save on commonly used products. Most people aren't aware of how easy and cheap it is to make many processed foods such as nut milk, granola, dehydrated fruits, etc. Even household cleaners can be made using common products and they can be safer as well

How to Spot Fake Food When You Go Shopping

I admit that this topic almost sounds like a joke. But it should not be too difficult to realize that in general, many of us don't realize that much of what is commonly sold as "food" isn't really food. Some of this stuff is so denatured and chemically-processed that our bodies don't regard it as legitimate nutrition. Because of this deception, those who consume the most of these fake foods are undergoing advancing stages of malnutrition.

When sustained over longer periods of time, malnutrition weakens immunity, putting us at greater risk of chronic diseases, systemic inflammation, and rapid aging. Earlier we discussed the "Paradox of Evolving" and what happens when we continuously expose our bodies to a broad range of

29 | Chapter 3 — If It's About Money, Consider This

environmental stresses, many of which didn't even exist a half-century ago.

Fake food stresses the cellular integrity of our bodies. While we may derive some measure of taste and bulk to offset the pangs of hunger after not eating for a while, filling hungry bellies with fake food is actually worse than being hungry. So much of this stuff consists of empty calories, excess sugar, salt and fat, as well as drugs and chemicals masquerading as food. We are thus wasting the opportunity to experience proper nutrition by loading up instead on this crap.

Fake food gets massive advertising dollars from food processing corporations. Sweets and candy, cookies, chips, sodas, fast food restaurants, artificially colored and flavored novelties made from a base of processed corn, soybeans, wheat, and potatoes — It's insane what these advertisements have convinced people to eat!

When you go into a grocery store, do you make time to read food labels for nutritional content? It is a fact that most people eat the same dozen or so foods on a regular basis. It is also true that we establish many of our adult food habits at much younger ages and that we have retained an emotional attachment to certain foods because of lingering feelings associated with childhood experiences. As a child we did not read food labels.

Here's a simple experiment I want you to try. Next time you go to a full-service supermarket, find a manager or someone who knows what's going on and ask this question: "Excuse me, can you tell me where your health food section is located?"

Chances are you will receive a response such as, "Go to aisle six, half-way down on the left is the health food section."

Your second question is, "Well, if that is the *health* food section, what then is the rest of the store?" An honest response to that follow-up might be a shocker, "Oh, that's what Americans eat."

As part of our **30-Days to a New You** reboot, we're taking charge of what we put in our mouths and into the bellies of our children, who need us to get this right. Here are three simple steps to flip this to our advantage.

1) Get into the habit of reading all food labels. Develop your food-ingredient literacy. What is the significance of the amount of sugar, fiber, vitamins and fat content in this product? Did you know that ingredients should be listed in the order by which they appear in the greatest amount?

2) A simple but powerful rule applies here: If you can't pronounce it, it's probably not food. Many of these additives' names represent their chemical formula, such as: Allura Red AC (FDA Red #40 food coloring); acesulfame potassium (an artificial sweetener); ammonium polyphosphates (anti-caking agents); and ascorbic stearate (an antioxidant preservative) – You might get grossed out without even leaving those whose chemical names begin with an "A."

3) Establish a whole plant food-based nutritional lifestyle. You can't go wrong with fresh, locally-grown and organic produce from a farmer's market, community garden or your backyard. Remember always, old habits die hard, yet new habits are quick to start. Acquiring your groceries from fresh market sources is a great habit for you to initiate.

31 | Chapter 3 – If It's About Money, Consider This

Go to your refrigerator and your cupboards today and pull out all the processed foods, put them on the table and start to read and comprehend which chemical agents have sneaked into your family's diet. If you need to, pull out a magnifying glass to make sure that some manufacturer is not trying to trick you by making these labels difficult to read.

Get rid of fake food in your diet. You'll soon notice that your battle with systemic inflammation begins to turn in your favor. Most fake foods are acid-forming, and this is incompatible with your plans to avoid illness, stay off drugs, and live long.

Stop Wasting Money on Depleted Food

Processed food is almost always more expensive than making the fresh stuff yourself. When it is cheaper, most likely it is because the nutrients are not there in sufficient amounts to sustain health. A quart of ice cream can run $5 or more and still leave you quite unsatisfied after you've eaten the whole thing. This same amount of money invested in frozen bananas, strawberries, blueberries, etc. and then processed as a delicious creamy frozen dessert will feed you several times, make you feel satisfied, and boost your body's immune system. One of the primary causes of overweight and obesity is the overconsumption of nutrition-depleted, dead food.

Eating out is expensive unless you are feeding your family cheap, fast-food burgers, fries and soda—and you know how damaging that can be for your generalized health. Most restaurant food is more expensive than making it oneself at home. When you figure in the cost of feeding multiple family members, it becomes even more obvious that a lot of money becomes wasted on food that is often nutrient deficient. Too many of us have allowed the corporations to steal away our quality time which used to be committed to taking care of ourselves and family. Many people have gotten into the habit of eating out every day on their job or dining in expensive cafeterias. Get in the habit of carrying your food and snacks with you. Save money and eat higher quality.

I hope you are finding inspiration within this series of instructions to reinforce the **Get the Weight Off** program. By now, you should be able to see just how easy and practical this can become once one has reset many of the basic habits that we've carried for decades, which have led to a poor nutritional outcome. Go to the New Conscious Rasta Report 2012 and learn even more. Also, tell a friend or two or a dozen. You are a change-agent and it's time that we all get busy transforming our community into its greatest potential.

Chapter 4 – Childhood and Teen Obesity

Seeds Sown for Future Crises

As difficult as it is to get many members of this society to acknowledge that we have a major problem with overweight and obesity, there is one area where the evidence of crisis is rising very rapidly, and that is the special problem of excess weight among children and teens. Many adults are overweight due to emotional problems brought about because of earlier psychological trauma or as a maladaptive response to anxiety and the burden of everyday existence. The youngest overweight children do not have the experience of psychic injury and are yet too young to carry multiple societal burdens. By the time our youth reach their teenage years and start to develop autonomous life patterns, we had better make sure, as their parents, that we have shown them the pathway towards their own best decision-making about such critical areas as their health. The fact is that their parents' generation made most overweight children that way.

Let's look at some of the disturbing facts about the rise of this trend within our children. After examining these often-shocking facts about childhood and teen obesity, let us then go into our own experienced, creative, problem-solving mode and bring about some *practical* solutions:

Shocking Facts about Child and Teen Obesity

These are some disturbing statistics published by the federal government regarding child and teen obesity:

- Obesity is particularly a problem among low-income preschool children with 1 in 7 preschoolers already medically diagnosed as obese;

- States which have the highest rates of obese children age 2-4 include: Massachusetts, New Jersey, Maryland, Virginia, Kentucky, Texas, South Dakota, Oregon, and California;

- Among teenage boys in the U.S. obesity rates increased over the past two decades: among Hispanic boys from 11.6% to 16.7% (43% growth of incidence); Black males from 10.7% to 19.8% (85% growth of incidence); and among Whites from 14.1% to 26.8% (90% growth of incidence)

- Among teenage girls in the U.S. obesity rates grew in the past two decades: among Hispanic girls from 8.9% to 14.5% (63% growth of incidence); Black females from 16.3% to 29.2% (79% growth of incidence); and among Whites from 13.4% to 17.4% (30% growth of incidence)

- One can project these figures out over the next two decades and beyond and see that this crisis will be getting much, much worse if we do not change this trend immediately.

Factors Contributing to the Growing Epidemic of Fat Children

According to the **American Academy of Child & Adolescent Psychiatry**, factors which cause obesity among youth include:

- **Poor eating habits** – There is a large contribution to this factor by mass media marketing of junk food, fast food and highly processed foods.

35 | Chapter 4 – Childhood and Teen Obesity

- **Overeating or binging** – This is largely due to the low nutrient content of foods consumed.

- **Lack of exercise** – This is a result of an increasingly sedentary lifestyle, much due to the impact of being tethered to electronic entertainment.

- **A family history of obesity** – Contrary to what many families have been told, the commonality of overweight within the family is NOT about genes. It is about habits and traditions that run in families.

- **Congenital factors** – This could largely be due to the result of gestational issues, injury in the womb, which may be because of a toxic environment around the pregnancy.

- **Pharmaceutical medications** – We are living in a drugged-out nation, over-medicated society. Now they are overdosing our children.

- **Stressful life changes** – Many children are experiencing instability within the family and bullying at school or throughout the society.

- **Low self-esteem** – Too many children are not being educated and encouraged toward being creative and feeling confident.

- **Depression or other emotional problems** – Many young people today are anxious about their future within the larger society which can lead to depression, and a deficit of optimism.

Are Your Children What *You* Eat?

What foods are America's obese children eating? – For the most part, the same foods (and portions) that overweight parents are eating. For overweight eaters there is an excess of: fat, sugar and salt, highly-processed foods, hormones and steroids in animal fats, endocrine-disrupting chemicals (EDC's) in the foods, and diets that are severely lacking in the most critical nutrients, such as fiber, vitamins, minerals, enzymes, complex carbohydrates, and essential fatty acids.

Some of the top junk food and fast food offenders, which contribute significantly to the obesity crisis are: donuts, potato chips, French fries, other fried foods, soda, red meat, bacon, processed meats containing nitrates, white flour products, whole milk products, salad dressings, margarine, hormones within the meat, pizza, candy, as well as soft drinks containing high amounts of sugar and fructose corn syrup.

The Family Meal – Is S.A.D. the Best You Can Do?

We often rail about the poor standard of health caused by the Standard American Diet (S.A.D.). Within this wealthy nation, we have a strange phenomenon compared to less-wealthy nations: elsewhere poverty is associated with being underweight while in the U.S. poverty is associated with overweight and medical problems associated with obesity. Much of this is because inexpensive, cheap food in the U.S. is nutrient-deficient, fatty, compromised by chemical additives and disproportionately distributed among poorer neighborhoods.

37 | Chapter 4 – Childhood and Teen Obesity

Whole families are in patterns of poor eating habits. The sit-down family meal is becoming rare in many households with too many children eating in front of the television, which is feeding them poor habits and nutrition ideas all the while. All people, including children, are eating too fast and not allowing their food to be chewed sufficiently for proper digestion. An average household refrigerator is stuffed with toxic agents of disorder and malnutrition. Not enough families emphasize drinking purified water in sufficient amounts to prevent the many problems associated with dehydration, even impacting youth.

The Sedentary Child in American Society

We have acknowledged the trend of youth today to spend too much time watching television, playing electronic games, surfing the Internet, deep into their so-called "smartphones" and other non-physical activities, to include long hours sitting in classrooms. Many schools are cutting back on physical education programs that engage our children in exercise. The children who most engage this sedentary lifestyle, combined with the poor food choices promoted within this society are the most at risk for the problems of overweight and obesity. Beyond the sedentary aspect of many of these activities, they also lead to isolation and disconnection from the larger social environment. In previous generations youth from the U.S. excelled in the world of sports far above other nations. That physical advantage eroded away because of the trend among American youth to spend so much time in non-physical activities and avoiding sports competition.

Changing Household Habits

The primary place where we will resolve the child and teen obesity crisis is within the household, and parents and grandparents of these children will direct this turnaround. We cannot and should not rely on government agencies and profit-driven businesses to be responsible for a change; the reasons for their unreliability are too many to mention in this brief article. Some of the things we can do within our homes include:

- Cutting down or cutting out the excessive time put into electronic entertainment;

- Keeping junk foods, sodas, and highly processed foods out of the house;

- Drinking water in sufficient amounts to be a compliment to health;

- Keeping a large bowl of fresh and tasty fruit in view in the kitchen or dining room as well as cleaned and cut fruits and veggies available for quick snacks;

- Bring fresh vegetables to the table daily, prepared healthy;

- Have a family time every week, or even every day, to engage in exercise, play, beach time, gardening, yoga or other physical activity which engages their cardiovascular system.

Keeping Our Youth Enthusiastic About Life

So much of what we're describing regarding this emerging crisis of child and teen obesity is related to low self-esteem, diminishing social and economic opportunities for the future, the infection of the minds of youth with corrupted ideas from the *merchants of cultural death* and the instability of the family as a basic survival unit. Solutions to this crisis will be complex, and these trends won't be easy to redirect toward the more positive outcome. Nonetheless, this is a time that challenges our creative, practical and inspirational talents or skills. We have proven in previous times of great crisis that yes, we are resourceful and yes, we can do miracles through commitments.

Within our youth we've got much work to do to develop a powerful sense of their self-worth, esteem, appreciation of their individuality, and unique talents. In areas of artistic expression, there is a great historical record of the youth's exceptionality. Athletics is another area where we can invest a great measure toward a productive outcome. We must be bold enough to get our young people out of the grasp of the merchants of cultural death and to explain to them the many ironies and contradictions of this society and world that they are inheriting. We must find creative ways to teach our youth critical decision-making at the earliest age possible, such as which snack would they like to choose that is healthiest for them (a tactic which I used with my daughters as early as three years of age)?

We've often heard and agree with the statement: "No nation can rise any higher than the status of its women." Then again what of a nation, especially a *wealthy* nation, that is producing children that are 1) less wealthy, 2) less educated, and 3) less *healthy* than their parent's generation? As much as we see the consequences of these areas as they impact the general population, it doesn't take rocket science to realize that it's going to get much worse decades from now according to the current trend. Because we have seen this crisis many years before it is fully actualized, we must now make critical decisions as to where we will invest resources to bring about the optimal condition for our children and future generations to live to their fullest potential.

Chapter 5 – A Radical New Concept of "Dieting"

Why I Don't Advocate Dieting

Have you noticed how many people strive to reduce their weight by dieting only to fail consistently? How is it that most profit-driven diet businesses have such a terrible record of freeing their clients from needing their services within a reasonable period? These simple steps we are sharing each day allow us to establish new habits that transform our healthy lifestyle.

According to PR Web, the U.S. weight loss market was worth over $60 billion in 2009 and growing at a rate of about 3%, despite the impact of the recession on household budgets. It has is reported that people are spending thousands, tens of thousands, and as much as $100,000 on various weight loss schemes, yet still finding themselves overweight, obese and frustrated after each experience. An online inquiry via a search engine using the words "weight loss" brings up a never-ending list of resources which are contradictory, ineffective and painful to employ.

I want to share a radical new concept of "dieting" which I am convinced will assist you to transform your body and achieve your goal within a reasonable time and *without dieting*.

One of the primary reasons for diet failure is because people associate weight reduction with starvation, caloric restriction, and punishing exercise. As well, there is a failure to consider that such deprivations are *not what the body needs*. We should seek to acquire a naturally-balanced weight within what health advocates call *homeostasis*.

Despite diet starvation and the constant discomfort that it brings, year after year people persist in this frustrating "dance with the devil." People find themselves caught up in an endless merry-go-round of weight loss supplements, bizarre diet schemes, distracting TV commercials, ineffective drugging – all the while become ever more frustrated, anxious, angry and resenting those whose physics spare them endless cycles of dancing with this devil called dieting.

Counting Calories is Pointless and Distracting

Counting calories is largely a waste of your time and attention, although it is one of the most common techniques used by weight loss profiteers. By counting calories, the dieter believes that reducing weight is merely a simple mathematical equation of subtraction. It's a stupid and pointless strategy largely for the following reasons:

- The idea of one healthy standard of daily calorie consumption doesn't take into consideration of key distinctions in our physiology and lifestyle – there is no one-size-fits-all model;

- Calories come in a wide variety of concentrations. Consuming 300 calories of highly-nutritional organic spinach compared to 300 calories of *fiberless* lean meat will produce a completely different health outcome;

- Depending on the overall quality of nutrition that the body wisely senses, "burning calories" can have different rates of

43 | Chapter 5 — A Radical New Concept of "Dieting"

efficiency because key vitamins, minerals, enzymes and other catalytic agents are necessary to the efficiency of producing cellular energy;

- Calorie counting simply doesn't work well for the majority of those who try it.

When the body senses that starvation is imminent due to caloric restriction it shifts to energy-conserving metabolism and burns calories at a much slower rate. As such, exercise often doesn't produce an expected shedding of fat for fuel (*ketosis*) despite calorie-burning mathematical formulas constantly being pursued by those caught up in weight loss schemes.

Additionally, many people exist in a constant state of malnutrition. You could be lacking in the seven critical nutrient classes: vitamins, minerals, protein (amino acids), carbohydrates, enzymes, essential fatty acids, *and* water. Because your body is starving for these key nutrients, excess food in the form of inaccessible calories, is converted to fat which stores throughout the body.

The body uses and stores energy in three forms: 1) blood sugar (glucose); 2) glycogen (stored in limited amounts within the liver and muscles for easy access to energy); and 3) body fat (excess glycogen stores in limitless amounts as fat). Key to properly metabolizing fat is that there are essential vitamins and minerals which, along with active enzymes, allow efficient conversion of energy reserves to metabolism, wherein we are generating energy through cell mitochondria (little sugar-burning engines within each cell).

Implement the three following instructions into your plan for creating space for diet-less weight reduction:

1) Instead of focusing on confusing mathematics centered around counting calories, focus instead on getting the widest spectrum of the eight critical nutrient classes we need to remain healthy; get them in the highest concentration available and in the most digestible form.

2) Because high caliber superfoods with maximum nutrient density contribute so much more to dietary integrity, you can get by with eating less while still feeling satisfied. One of the keys to reaching satiation is to chew your food completely. Slow your roll and count anywhere from 32 to 48 chews before you swallow. Liquifying your food before swallowing significantly increases digestibility.

3) Fresh, fully-ripened seasonal fruits are perfect for getting your maximum healthy on. Eating local fruit within the natural rhythm of the seasons brings us into harmony with Nature. If you ever lived with fruit trees, you know very well the benefits of eating fresh plums, cherries, grapes, figs, apples, or oranges when these trees are at their peak of harvest. The fact is that humans primarily evolved as fruit eaters.

The Digestive System is Smarter Than You Think

WE are frequently told that we *consciously* engage only from 5% to 15% of our brain as sentient humans. The fact is that we engage 100% of our brain – because *it is our brain* and we need to appreciate the greater function of brain activity that is constantly taking place. The "autonomic nervous system" (ANS) operates outside of our conscious thought process and is responsible for controlling *visceral functions* of the body such

45 | Chapter 5 – A Radical New Concept of "Dieting"

as heart rate, digestion, respiration, salivation, perspiration, urination, sexual arousal and other critical body functions.[1]

There is an extensive neural sensing network which makes up our digestive system, including:

- Visual, olfactory and gustatory sensory perception of the quality of food through the sight, smell and taste of the food;

- Triggers within the mouth to stimulate saliva production and the enzyme amylase, which processes complex carbohydrates (polysaccharides) into simple sugars (disaccharides, or maltose);

- Satiation mechanisms which give us a sense of fullness when the stomach has reached a certain capacity or when we have eaten for a length of time (20 minutes or more);

- The hormone *cholecystokinin* is produced by the digestive system and signals the brain when we've eaten. When dieting, the stomach counterbalances reduced food intake by cutting back on the release of this hormone, encouraging one to return to overeating after dieting;

- Sensors to detect the fat content of a meal, triggering the production of human pancreatic lipase (HPL) which then catalyzes fats for breakdown into amino acids;

---

[1] Definition of Autonomic Nervous System from Wikipedia.org

- Other sensors in the stomach can detect glucose (sugar), carbohydrates, proteins, enzymes, minerals, alcohol, hydration, heat, bacterial toxins, and so forth.

- Nerve cells in the gut use both electrical (nervous) and hormonal (serotonin) signaling to tell the brain a mass of details about the food we are consuming. We find that there are "over 100 billion neurons in the human gut" functioning within signaling systems."[2]

How the Body Switches to High-Efficiency

Not only does our digestive-brain communication process radically shift during nutritional deficiency *or* abundance, but in the presence of starvation, the body compensates by switching to a high-efficiency model. Those of us who have experienced fasting realize that at a certain point we will become constipated as the body retains the last of the food in the intestinal tract toward the aim of extracting whatever nutrients it can access. This example points out why so many malnourished people experience recurrent constipation even though they have a mass of "food" still within the lower intestine. A buildup of impacted fecal mass is what's often behind that bulging stomach syndrome which is plaguing so many members of wealthy, overfed societies.

When the body senses that starvation is imminent due to caloric restriction it shifts to an energy-conserving metabolism and burns calories at a significantly slower rate. As such, exercise doesn't produce an expected burning of fat for fuel (*ketosis*) despite calorie-burning mathematical formulae

---

[2] Our Second Brain: The Stomach, from Psychology Today, May 1, 1999

47 | Chapter 5 – A Radical New Concept of "Dieting"

constantly being pursued by those caught up in weight loss trends.

Additionally, many people exist in a constant state of malnutrition. Lacking in the seven critical nutrient classes: vitamins, minerals, protein (amino acids), carbohydrates, enzymes, essential fatty acids, *and* water. Because the body senses that it is starving for these key nutrients, extra consumed food in the form of inaccessible calories, is converted to fats which store throughout the body.

The body uses and stores energy in three forms: 1) blood sugar (glucose); 2) glycogen (stored in limited amounts within the liver and muscles for easy access to energy); and 3) body fat (excess glycogen stores in limitless amounts as fat). The key to properly metabolizing fat is that there are essential vitamins and minerals which, along with living enzymes, allow efficient conversion of these energy reserves to metabolism, wherein we are generating energy through cell mitochondria (little sugar-burning engines within each cell).

With insufficient access to critical nutrients, we experience a degree of starvation which triggers the body to switch to the *logic of efficiency*, which is the mechanism behind the frustrating failure of "dieting" for weight reduction. As well, this logic is also why most people rapidly put back on the excess weight when their "diet" fails.

Lose Weight" While Eating Growth Hormones?

A lot of very bad weight loss propaganda persists throughout society. Much of this is simply incomplete research, but a degree of it must be regarded as *deliberate* disinformation to keep a captive population stupid enough to keep on buying into the same set of ineffective tactics. People are most often advised to use low-fat dairy products, eat lean meat, or switch from red meats to poultry toward the aim of rebalancing the metabolic system.

Because high amounts of chemicals are commonly added to the diets of these feed animals, one can be eating less meat-derived calories while still consuming substances that are *intended* to cause rapid and sustained weight gain within the animal. With the presence of unnatural amounts of growth hormones, estrogenic chemicals, antibiotics, and steroids within these foods, it is a *foolish and futile strategy* to attempt to reduce the weight by continuing to eat food that generates weight gain.

Full-Spectrum Hyper Nutrition to the Rescue

What is "full-spectrum hyper nutrition?"

Our body's cellular structure, organic and systemic functions require a spectrum of key nutrients to be healthy and to thrive. These key nutrients are hydration, vitamins, minerals, protein (amino acids), carbohydrates, essential fatty acids, fiber, and active enzymes.

Within this Reboot regime, our goal is to supply excessive amounts of the previously-mentioned eight critical classes of nutrients, in the most bio-available delivery-method possible, toward the aim of Full-Spectrum Hyper Nutrition. When this accomplished in an eating style where one requires no more than 1000 to 1500 calories per day, then beneficial changes

49 | Chapter 5 — A Radical New Concept of "Dieting"

begin to take place; and I hope you recall that in our strategy for weight reduction, we do not rely on counting calories.

To maximize our strategies for creating perfect health, we've developed multiple strategies:

- We target pathological conditions which set up disease and disorder for disruption and elimination. The root of disease is called "pathogenesis," and we base our system of nutrition-based medicine on preventing the creation of disease. Elimination of the roots of disease is known as "functional medicine."

- Once we've eliminated these underlying conditions, diseases and disorders with their accompanying symptoms cease to manifest. Overweight and obesity are symptoms of malnutrition; therefore in combatting excess weight, we concentrate on full-spectrum hyper nutrition to reverse malnutrition.

- Corrective processes are given more energy during our nightly restoration cycle of sleep. It is during sleep that sustained healing, repairing and rejuvenation take place. This period of sleep-restoration is known as senescence.

- Because the body is no longer stressed and diverting energy to extensive restoration, we now have more energy available for other needed cellular processes. This energy will manifest in other parts of our metabolism, resulting in increasingly adaptive physiological activity.

- Once these healing processes accomplished in nightly maintenance are complete, the body uses this extra energy for rejuvenation as it goes through its natural cycle replacing all 50 trillion cells over 11 months' time, restoring optimal function to each of the body's organic systems.

The role of full-spectrum hyper nutrition during all these stages of healing is critical. Because we have focused so intensely on providing this basis, we can get the maximum benefit of the body's natural processes for healing and revitalizing itself.

Here are a few simple steps to achieve full-spectrum hyper nutrition:

1) Read, study and comprehend the critical importance of consuming foods which best deliver the hydration, vitamins, minerals, proteins (amino acids), essential fatty acids, active enzymes, complex carbohydrates, and fiber that our body needs for full-spectrum nutrition.
2) Incorporate as many superfoods into the diet as possible. These are foods which contain the highest concentration of these essential nutrients in the most bio-available delivery available.
3) Don't undermine your strategy for hyper nutrition by consuming junk foods, dead foods and a high amount of acid-forming foods. There is a simple understanding here that "you are what you eat." Make sure you are not eating considerable amounts of junk and death if you intend to avoid becoming dead junk.

Full-spectrum hyper nutrition – yeah, it may sound like a mouthful of science. With Living Superfood, we strive to make it tasty, and the research we put into hyper nutrition can very

51 | Chapter 5 — A Radical New Concept of "Dieting"

well save your life and dramatically improve the health and well-being of your entire family.

Burn Body Fat Without Starving

So, the goal is to restore proper nutrition to our lifestyle, rid ourselves of the symptoms of malnutrition, repair all the damage, raise our energy level and return to the stage of our life when we were youthful and healthy. Let's do as much of the following as possible to succeed in this strategy:

- Increase your hydration level by drinking the proper amount of high-quality water;

- Gain access to the seven critical nutrients by consuming excessive amounts of these elements from whole-plant-based diets. These diets work best-using living foods (not enzyme depleted), grown organically (much more nutrient dense), fresh and locally grown (from your garden is ideal). These fresh foods then need to be prepared in ways that 1) do not damage the nutrients, and 2) do not introduce toxicity into the food—this we best accomplish with raw superfoods;

- Include in your regime regular detoxification and fasting to clean out the bowels and allow for higher efficiency of nutrient absorption from the intestinal tract;

- Chew your food slowly allowing digestive enzymes to do the work for which they are intended. Ideally, food should be chewed from 32-48 times, until it is completely liquefied, before swallowing. Additionally, do not "wash your food down" with any beverage while eating. If your mouth becomes too dry to properly salivate while eating, pause for a few minutes and take small sips of no more than a tablespoon of water at a time until ready to proceed again;

- Eat smaller meals spaced out throughout the day, allowing your digestive system to function at a higher efficiency by not being overwhelmed, which produces "The Itis" condition which makes one sleepy after eating a particularly obnoxious meal;

- Stop eating foods that have become contaminated with growth hormones, steroids, antibiotics, uric acid, etc.—in other words, stop eating meat;

- Juicing is the optimal way to get access to nutrients, green juicing is the best for weight reduction because of its role in significantly increasing the blood's capacity for carrying the oxygen needed for metabolism to function at its optimal level;

- Keep moving throughout the day, especially if you have a sedentary job. Try one or more of the following: a brisk morning walk, stretching, yoga or working out with hand weights before breakfast, parking your car away from your work entrance or shopping destination, isometric exercises, vigorous activity while cleaning the home, washing your own car, mowing your own lawn, working in the garden, and TURNING OFF THE TELEVISION. All of these are ways in which the natural cycle of burning of stored up energy take place;

- Consume nothing but water and fresh fruit before noon each day. Also, be careful with fruit juices as some juices

Chapter 5 — A Radical New Concept of "Dieting"

contain too high amounts of fructose (fruit sugar) to allow us to get to ketosis. Bottled, pasteurized juices are not bad but are enzyme-depleted because of the heat of pasteurization. If you use them, mix them with something that does contain living enzymes (enzymes are not living, but their activation is dependent upon them not being heated beyond a certain critical temperature, usually about 125 degrees Fahrenheit or less);

- Don't eat after sundown or at least four hours before going to sleep.

In contrast to much of what is a commonly-held belief about body weight management, you likely will agree that this is a radical way of looking at "dieting." The facts are there to confirm or deny the authenticity of this information that I've shared. I know that this works because I experienced the transformation, reducing my weight by 35 lbs. from my lifetime high of 180 and keeping it now at its natural low.

During one 28-day detoxification fast, I witnessed a reduction in my weight from 176 pounds to 150, a decline of 16% of my body weight. I did engage in extensive water fasting and colon cleansing during that time which I caution *may be too much* for the novice to fasting detoxification.

Go to the website **GetTheWeightOff.info** and get on board. You don't want to miss THIS train — Get on board before it leaves the station.

Chapter 6 – Women's Weight and "The Burden"

What Do the Numbers Say?

Statistics can be a myriad of things. Statistics can be misleading when used for political or financial exploitation. Statistics can be frightening, too often leading to a "deer in the headlights" response where a person is unable to respond to the shock which can result from "statistical overload." Far too many people are overwhelmed by numbers and will quickly close off their reasoning mind when statistics are used to make key points of reference.

For some, statistics are a necessary foundation upon which they can gauge the proper direction toward which to turn. Some of us are so concerned with making the best decisions that we draw toward statistical measurement as another analytical resource toward empowerment.

The trend toward overweight and obesity in the U.S., as well as other developed nations, is shocking. The following data on obesity trends come from the CDC online site, the Department of Health and Human Services, and online resources related to overweight and obesity:

- In 2009-2010, 78 million ages 20 and above were obese in the U.S., 35.7% of the adult population; the majority were women; [In updating this statistic, according to the JAMA Journal, the obesity rate for American adults increased to 39.6% for the years 2015-2016.]

55 | Chapter 6 – Women's Weight and "The Burden"

- Obesity is overweight with resultant medical conditions which include (but are not limited to) cardiovascular diseases, stroke, diabetes, cancer, infertility and premature death;

- Obesity affects U.S. Blacks at the highest rate over other ethnic groups;

- In the general population higher income equates to lower rates of obesity; for Blacks and Hispanic men, obesity rates are higher for those with higher income;

- African American women have the highest rates of overweight or obesity compared to other groups with estimates for black women over the age of 18 as high as 30.4% overweight and an additional 54% obese;

- More than 80% of people with Type 2 diabetes are overweight

- Black women have more than double the likelihood of early death from heart disease and stroke compared to Whites. The same is true for men.

Overweight and obesity is primarily a consequence of – symptomatic of several lifestyle factors, including:

- Consuming excess calories for one's physical activity engaged daily;

- The sedentary lifestyle, lack of exercise, etc.;

- Consuming a high percentage of animal protein for daily caloric input;

- Excessive amounts of LDL (low-density lipoprotein, the bad cholesterol) in the diet;

- Consuming foods contaminated with growth hormones, steroids, antibiotics;

- Inflammation due to consuming high amounts of acidic foods;

- Metabolic disorder (the body's mechanism for burning fuel has gone out of order);

- Congenital factors (genetic or in-utero injury);

- Dramatic alteration in hormone function, such as the transition to menopause;

- Low nutritional quality of food consumed and resultant intense food cravings.

What I am hearing from many working women is that they feel constrained by their job schedule, commuting time, personal responsibilities, all combining with household chores, and are thus finding it too inconvenient to spend time shopping for and preparing the healthiest food. Therefore, fast food industries step up to fill a critical need in these women's lives to provide a source of quick, tasty and inexpensive food.

A problem arises when the nutritional quality of fast food declines as it is made quicker and cheaper. Many of the techniques used to make such food palatable to the taste buds further compromise the integrity of the food. Fast food is excessively fatty, salty, sugary, with artificial ingredients, as well as containing toxic additives, such as MSG (monosodium

57 | Chapter 6 – Women's Weight and "The Burden"

glutamate) which are known to damage the body the more of it we eat. Fast food favorites include substances known to raise the risk of cancer, such as *acrylic* amide. Some people are eating this toxic fast food more than ten times a week.

Reversing Obesity-Related Disease

Primary among our strategies toward reversing the trends which are leading to greater numbers of overweight and obese women within this society must be an effort to lessen the *burden* that women are carrying. The rate at which women are represented within the corporate labor force is greater than it has ever been. With the current level of social and economic demand on those struggling within an increasingly expensive urban landscape, we much change our habits to remain creative and committed. We must be willing to let certain highly-valued aspects of our lives go so that we can restore a functional community environment that supports women.

Habits will have to change. We need to suppress material desires towards the greater fulfillment of spiritual, psychological and cultural values. We can override selfish motives and replace them with those that serve family, community, and humanity. Greater attention to the true needs of women will have to become a priority of the larger community, especially among men.

Here are a few suggestions for women to push the weight of The Burden out of your pathway to vitality, health, and longevity:

1. Shift some of your daily activities to the early morning. If you are up past sundown, then allocate your time so that you can sleep earlier and arise at or before dawn. Sunrise is truly a magical time of the day, and you should capture some of its magical energy for your fulfillment.

2. Prepare your lunch at home and take with you to work. Fixing our own lunch is not only great for health reasons, but the creativity which goes into creating a beautiful lunch will be matched by the expressions of fellow workers when they see your craft. Take a little extra food with you and use it to impress your fellow workers.

3. If you have a long or stressful commute to work, fill that time with life-affirming audio recordings. You can make them yourself, purchase audio books or collect and trade motivational recordings. It's good to remind ourselves of our self-worth and value constantly.

4. Learn breathing techniques that can use to de-stress in a minute or two. There are times during your work day when others simply get on your nerves. If you don't have a deliberate technique to rid yourself of the toxic poison from such encounters, it will build up inside of you and find a way to show its displeasure. Re-channel the stress into something beneficial.

5. Eat small meals throughout the day instead of 2 to 3 large meals. Light eating lessens the load on the digestive tract, especially the pancreas, and lessens the risk of overweight, obesity, and diabetes. As well this helps to keep the energy balanced throughout the day so that there'll be no need for a toxic energy drink to get through the afternoon.

59 | Chapter 6 – Women's Weight and "The Burden"

6. Create or join a circle of mutual support at work as well as outside of the work environment. Join a book club, study group, women's circle, camping organization, sports team or some other function which allows you a chance to grow creatively outside of your employment.

7. Pick up at least one art or handcraft. It is essential that you have a chance to show your feminine creativity. Arts, crafts, music, poetry, and dance are all outlets for expelling stress.

8. Change your favorite foods to healthier means of preparation. Pizza can be made raw with a flax crust, homemade sauce, layered marinated vegetables, fruits, nut cheese, and mushrooms. We can reinvent virtually any meal as healthy nutrition. Again, be creative and experiment.

9. Allow 15 minutes a day to have a good brisk walk or bike ride. A good round of cardiovascular stimulation is critical toward longevity, hormone balance, and strong bones. The endorphins released during a stimulating round of exercise work magic throughout the system.

10. Enjoy a period of complete silence at times during each day. With all the unwelcome news, false values, distracting trivia and other background noise that is happening within our environment, sometimes you have to create an oasis of silence. Learn to recognize and take counsel from that still small voice of intuition deep within your soul.

11. Smile. Smile and laugh often. Volunteer wonderful energy and compassion for everyone you meet. It is no surprise that people infected with your exuberance and enthusiasm

are quick to reciprocate and do their best to be happy along with you. Be an agent of good feelings.

12. Drink more water. Flush the toxins from your body constantly.

13. Buy a set of quality supplements to make sure you are getting enough key nutrients for the complex systems of your body to function properly. This includes vitamins, minerals, enzymes, amino acids, essential fatty acids and probiotics. If you can, always strive to obtain these critical nutrients from fresh, locally grown, organic vegetables and fruits. Insure that you are not starving your body from what it truly needs to be healthy.

14. Have a plan for keeping your health in order. You must plan your lifelong health as if you were planning to build a small business. Without such a plan, you run the danger of randomly doing whatever is convenient, only to find that one day you are paying for mistakes that have been occurring for many years. Plan to live a long and vital life, free from dependence on pharmaceutical drugs. Plan to be the healthiest of your circle, your family or your workplace.

15. Keep on researching and studying what it takes to have such great health. Your obligation is to yourself to have the best possible outcome in your life. Take full responsibility for continued education and growth. Think of your health as an advanced graduate degree for which you are committing your entire life to achieve at its highest level. A lifelong pursuit of knowledge is also a strong factor to avoid the debilitation of mental decline in our senior years.

There is a great reason to be optimistic when one has a strong plan for success. It is likely that you have been feeling burdened with pressures from home duties, relationships, work-related stress and the ever-increasing set of demands upon your person. It is time to formulate a new plan. Get excited about the possibilities which lie ahead. Identify every resource and advantage for which Creation has blessed you. Remember that a "journey of a thousand miles" does indeed begin with one step. It is when one is stepping, stepping, stepping in a rhythm that you are assured of not only making your destination but knowing when you will arrive.

More Time in Your Days; More Days in Your Life

Among the many discussions I engage with people who want to establish the set of habits needed to sustain an ultimate nutrition lifestyle, they consistently raise one roadblock. With so many already-existing commitments on their time, people say they can't commit time for daily food preparation.

Let me make one point clear, and I've proven this over the course of 40 years of hands-on experience: The vegan lifestyle creates more time in your life than it costs to maintain. You are going to want to trust that I am sharing a powerful truth that I've proven through decades of experience and study.

Others report what I have experienced since going 98% raw vegan over the past 8 ½ years. Raw vegans reduce the need for sleep-repairing by two hours a day on average. For most people, it's hard to imagine converting from the **Standard American Diet** style of eating, which most have adopted, to something as radical as raw-vegan-organic-superfood with detoxing.

As an additional bonus, that feeling of drowsiness we refer to as "The Itis" which you get after eating a large meal disappears when you're not suffering the pro-inflammatory condition called *digestive leukocytosis*, the result of eating lifeless food. As such, the quality of your waking time improves as well.

With Living Superfood, you can recover two extra hours a day, and this adds up to 14 hours a week, over 30 days a year – just by eating smarter. Further, considering the conclusions in my book **LIVING SUPERFOOD LONGEVITY**, these strategies should lengthen life expectancy above "average" by a consistent 30 years.

The advantage which I am presenting to you with Living Superfood is that this lifestyle adds 8.3% more time to your days and this compounds to 42% more days for your superfood-extended lifespan. What did I say: 33.3 extra days per year, multiplied by 30 extra years for your life, equals 910 extra days created over the course of the extended lifespan! Add that time to the 10,957 days of your extended life expectancy. Do you think it wise that you would complain that you "don't have time" to **switch to daily habits that will add 42% more high-quality time to your entire life?!!**

Let's make this time. Here are three simple steps for you to start this work TODAY.

1) Take an hour away from your late-night activities and shift this time to early morning. Use this hour to prepare two Living Superfood dishes in enough quantity to last for three days,

63 | Chapter 6 — Women's Weight and "The Burden"

about six servings per person. Raw vegan food is best when eaten within 60 hours after preparation, or 2-3 days. Set aside one hour later in the day to prepare two additional superfood dishes. Constantly explore new recipes, so you don't get bored and undernourished by eating the same foods over and over. You can squeeze in a quick and healthy juice or smoothie during the middle of the day as well.

2) Get a set of glass containers for storing your highly nutritious food. Glass keeps superfood more stable and prevents toxic plastic molecules from leaching into the food and wreaking havoc with your hormones.

3) Find a partner or several others with which to collaborate. Make larger proportions and share them with family, co-workers, and those in your support group. Along with your group, plan to host weekly, bi-weekly or monthly healthy food meetups and vegan potlucks. At these feasts, you can share recipes and otherwise show support for the common mission.

You may have often heard it said that "time lost can't be recovered." Living Superfood proves that this statement is not absolute. Use all these techniques you are learning this month; you have new tools for managing, manufacturing and mastering the essence of time. Every time we are together I want to affirm this with you: **Live long, love strong and prosper.**

Get into action with our **Get the Weight Off 30-Day Program**. You won't regret taking on this transforming challenge.

Chapter 7 – Four Stages of Healing

I love talking about the miracle of *Living Superfood*™. I frequently initiate conversations on the topic with the words "What if..." I do my best to stimulate people's imagination and to challenge them to project themselves in a younger state. This is best accomplished by tapping their memory of what their physical state was at half their current chronological age. This works well with most people yet sometimes a person's recollection of their body when younger is that of someone who was not healthy. This requires a different approach.

A key point here is that it requires a strong mental concept of a destination before we can truly imagine completing the journey. Within modern society people have gotten all too accustomed to poor health as a general standard. Many have come to perceive that upon reaching age 40 to 50 years it is expected that a person will be exhibiting some signs of age-related chronic disease.

We have been *taught* to accept pathological physical conditions as normal. Too often nowadays the following pessimistic outcomes are widely accepted: 1) that most adults will be taking some form of prescription drugs by middle age; 2) that seniors will be infirmed in some manner due to degenerative disorders; and 3) that excessive weight will never go away unless we starve ourselves into a miserable existence.

But, what if...?

What if this devolution into degenerating health were a consequence of a lifetime of poor judgments which could have

65 | Chapter 7 – Four Stages of Healing

been reversed had we known the outcome? What if we have reliable tools available to us at this point in history that allow life expectancies more than 90 or 100 years to become commonplace? What if the body was actually *designed* to be capable of repairing itself, restoring and rejuvenating one to the perception of invincibility which we felt when in the prime of our youth?

These "What if..." questions have been answered and I have wonderful news to report. I am living testament to the fact that the Fountain of Youth is real and in our possession. I've created a vehicle to promote it called **Living Superfood**. I am certainly *not* the only one in possession of this knowledge; it's spreading rapidly through certain segments of the conscious-eating population. Yet I acknowledge that I have been allotted a special set of insights that go beyond what others in this field have mastered.

So let's take this journey through the **Four Stages of Health** that you can reasonably expect to experience once you commit yourself to the discipline and mastery of this science I call *Full-Spectrum Hyper Nutrition*. It is time to imagine your miracle and to order it up right away. Let me explain to you just how it is expected to proceed.

Stage 1 – Removing the Underlying Cause of Disease

Most chronic diseases and disorders have underlying causes which follow consistent rules of body mechanics. When disease symptoms appear, something is missing or out of order, key components have malfunctioned, and the result is a diseased condition with resultant symptoms. The process is called *pathogenesis* (pathos = injury; genesis = creation). Among the primary causes of chronic disease is malnutrition, the result of deprivation within one or more of the primary classes of nutrients the body needs on a constant basis. Unconscious eating, junk food, fast food, the Standard American Diet (S.A.D.) and prolonged exposure to toxic chemicals within our food all make us vulnerable to malnutrition.

A very long list of malnutrition-related disorders that result in pathogenesis include (but most certainly are *not* limited to):

- **Vitamin deficiencies** – There are a spectrum of vitamins that are essential to proper functioning within the body's various systems. These include vitamins A, B3, B6, B9, B12, C, D, E and K. Most of these have multiple functions within the body, too numerous to list within this short outline. I must emphasize that each of these vitamins is worthy of further research and some are so vital that life cannot proceed without their presence.

  A diet that is deficient in one or more vitamins could result in the following pathological symptoms: poor vision, skin rashes, eczema, slow wound healing, nerve damage, cognitive dysfunction, soft bones, tooth loss, malabsorption of lipids (fat), blood clotting problems, scurvy, arthritis, weakened immune system, poor appetite, gastric upset, mental depression, inflammation, sores in the mouth, anemia, diarrhea, dementia, convulsions, tumor growth, psychiatric disorders, hair loss and much more.

67 | Chapter 7 – Four Stages of Healing

- **Protein deficiencies** – Proteins are the basic building block of all living materials. While it is largely mythology that one must eat meat to get protein, it is undeniable that vegetarians, along with meat eaters, can demonstrate symptoms of protein deficiency. It is generally recommended that from 25% to 40% of our diet should consist of calories derived from protein, the source of protein being equally as important as to the amount. Optimally, protein should be obtained from plant-based sources to avoid increased risk of cancer and cardiovascular disease from consuming extraordinary amounts of animal meat and dairy protein.

  Insufficient amounts of protein in the diet result in one or more of the following symptoms: fatigue, muscle wasting, bleeding gums, muscle cramping, cold extremities, hair loss, brittle fingernails, anorexia, loss of protein in critical organs (heart, intestines, stomach, kidneys, liver, etc.), impaired wound healing, and weakened immune system.

- **Mineral deficiencies** – Like vitamins, there is a long list of mineral nutrients that we must access daily in order to prevent symptoms of disease. Those needed in larger quantities include: calcium, magnesium, phosphorus, potassium, sodium, chlorine and sulfur. In addition, we require dozens of trace minerals (microminerals) including cobalt, copper, fluoride, iodine, iron, manganese, selenium and zinc. All these minerals can be supplemented but are best acquired by eating a wide diversity of plant-based foods along with spring water.

Symptoms of mineral deficiencies will vary depending on which minerals are missing, but could include: conditions affecting the skin, blood, neurological system, hair, gastrointestinal system, bones, nails, brain functioning and cardiovascular system. Specific disorders from insufficient amounts of *just one mineral* could include: anxiety, asthma, anorexia, birth defects, hardened arteries, mental disorders, hyperactivity, hypertension, hypothermia, insomnia, menstrual pain, muscle weakness, tremors, seizures, Sudden Infant Death, vertigo and more – and these result from *magnesium deficiency alone!* For sake of keeping this document brief I can't list all the symptoms of deficiency for all of the aforementioned minerals.

- **Amino acid deficiencies** – Amino acids are nitrogen-containing molecules which are the building blocks of proteins, of which living matter is composed. There are 20 different amino acids that are assembled into hundreds of thousands of enzymes, proteins, antibodies and hormones. Our bodies can synthesize about half of these amino acids while the other half must be obtained from dietary sources.

  Symptoms of amino acid deficiencies would be expected to cover the entire spectrum of functions within the body, to include: neurological and brain malfunction, skin rashes, celiac disease, autoimmune disorders, inflammation, depression and mood issues, weak immune system, digestive problems, chronic fatigue and metabolic disorder (syndrome X).

As you can see by the preceding four nutrient classes, I could continue extensively as I have only briefly covered half of 8

69 | Chapter 7 – Four Stages of Healing

critical nutrients needed on a constant basis to stay healthy. Given more space I could go on to show the critical needs and symptoms of deficiency for 4 other categories:

- Essential fatty acids – our critical need for the right type and balance of cholesterol;

- Hydration – water is a fundamental key to life;

- Enzymes – these catalytic agents facilitate molecular transformation;

- Dietary fiber – assures that our digestive tract can continue to process food for energy.

Let's move on. I think you certainly see the pattern by now. We can summarize by saying that ALL these nutrients are absolutely vital to our *wholistic* health and well-being. You now understand that deficiencies in ANY of them will result in significant disorder and pathogenesis of disease symptoms. As well, combinations of deficiencies guarantee that we will suffer chronic disease symptoms.

Stage 2 – Relief from Symptoms

It should seem logical that once the underlying condition of nutritional deficiencies is relieved that these diseases will no longer have a foundation for their manifestation. Our strategy to overcome these deficits is *Full-Spectrum Hyper Nutrition*, accessible through the dietary regime. This elevated nutrition lifestyle must be sustained long enough to allow the entire progression from deficiency-related disorder to pathogenesis, disease and resultant symptoms to reverse completely. As we rebalance each of these areas of critical nutrients, then with time the end results of numerous deficiencies disappear. The restorative process is progressive and thus begins to increase the rate at which we can redirect more energy toward healing and restoration. The more you have healed, the better you feel. These sustained good feelings create a feedback loop as you more rapidly progress toward a state called *homeostasis*, where body systems functionality is back in order.

I have now experienced living for more than 2 ½ years within the raw-vegan-organic-superfood-detoxification life. It has presented me with a golden opportunity to live relatively symptom free. On occasion when I do notice symptoms of disorder within my body, I quickly recognize the condition and devise a nutritional strategy to interrupt the underlying cause of pathogenesis.

My personal testament upon moving from vegan to Full-Spectrum Hyper Nutrition is remarkable. Symptoms such as tiredness upon wakening disappeared along with a nagging pain in my right shoulder which had plagued me for over a year. I recovered from the need for reading glasses. My weight stopped its roller coaster fluctuation between my quarterly fasts and has now stabilized 31 pounds lighter than I was when I began my last fast as a vegan. I gained all these benefits because I elevated my nutrition to that of a *raw superfoodist* while still maintaining seasonal detoxification fasting.

My cognitive functioning has improved, and I registered an increase in my tested IQ. These days I sleep only 5-6 hours at night yet wake up completely rejuvenated. Sexual libido has returned to the steamy level that it was in my late-twenties. Wounds heal much faster and I no longer "catch" colds or suffer nasal mucus plugs. I dropped the habit of hacking up mucus throughout the day. I rarely must deal with gastrointestinal stress, bloating and gas. My blood pressure last tested at 114 over 71 and I have not visited a doctor due to illness in over thirty years.

In other words, the symptoms of what people come to think of as normal aging have disappeared. I am younger than I was twenty years ago!

Stage 3 – Feeling the Energy Within

The next stage after the body corrects all the various disorders which had accumulated over the years is we become acutely aware of a tremendous reserve of energy that remains with us at the end of our nighttime restoration session. We don't have to rely on an alarm to awaken each morning. We feel grateful for life and enthusiastic about taking on our day and engaging critical tasks. We notice that we've begun to talk faster, walk faster, exercise more and feel more positively engaged within our world. Our internal energy generator now appears to be working to perfection. We are now functioning with a profound awareness that we are *energy beings*.

As we move through the day we encounter others to whom it appears obvious that something special is happening with us. They will comment on how clear our skin is, how young we look, how bright our attitude is and react as if they really enjoy being in our presence. We receive such positive feedback from social encounters that our respect for fellow humans increases and we project a loving appreciation for everything around us. Even those would-be detractors who deliberately try to hurt or hinder us are subject to our new stance of unrestricted possibilities. What was once perceived as an obstacle has now become an opportunity to validate our mastery of Life's greatest good.

In other words, we exist again as living gods and goddesses. I and many others believe this is the way that humans lived during a Golden Age of Civilization many thousands of years ago. This is how shamans, yogi, priests, sages, mystic women and men have continued to live within pristine environments and in monasteries around the world. This is how some farmers have known life over their decades of living closely within natural rhythms of life. You've now come to conscious awareness that this is a good life. When you are living a truly good life, you want others to experience it with you.

So, you may start to proselytize and to spread this good news. Be prepared, because people don't like to be reminded that they could be doing better. Most people will be resistant to your coaching and will present any handy excuse to justify staying within the same behavioral matrix that they have become familiar with. The people most in need of the very same healing which you are experiencing will resent you if you press too hard attempting to convince them to do what you've just done to liberate yourself. Eventually you'll learn to just relax and enjoy it for yourself. Later, when the student is ready, you the master will be recognized.

You must not allow pessimism within others to guide your life. Don't stop walking along this pathway. BE the example of that you would wish to propagate. Not everyone will acknowledge your transformation but enough will. Keep learning, growing

73 | Chapter 7 — Four Stages of Healing

and testing out new techniques while refining your ability to share your experience. Keep searching for even more advantages to this lifestyle. You will certainly be rewarded.

Among many rewards you will gain is increased awareness and reliability of *extra sensory* perception.

Just as you now register heightened perception within your five cognitive senses, your *intuition* will noticeably improve, and you will thus be better able to tap into your deep subconscious mind. Through intuition you can access your vast unconscious library and readily extract much wisdom which you have accumulated throughout the course of your life.

Additionally, your awareness of a sense of *clairvoyance* will become even more apparent. Through clairvoyance we occasionally find ourselves perceiving beyond limitations of time, space and personality. At times you'll surprise yourself with how you have come to *know* something that "common sense" might have told you that you shouldn't have possibly known. Such are the powers of a living god or goddess. Your phenomenal increase in radiant energy has brought you to the point that your Word now speaks into BE-ing that which needs to manifest.

You are now experiencing the Miracle of Life. So why not at this point order up a chance to revisit your youthful prime and live the second half of your life again anew? This time you have your current experience, wisdom and matured values to accompany you. This is the miracle of the Fountain of Youth.

Stage 4 – Rejuvenation

The adult human body contains between 50 and 70 *trillion* cells, each of which is replaced during a course of up to 11 months. As we age, there is a region within our DNA chromosomes which is called a *telomere* which shortens with the passage of time and thus prevents cells from replicating themselves with perfect copies. Aging is associated with DNA degeneration. Geneticists have traditionally regarded this process to be irreversible without intervention and much research has gone on to figure out ways to replenish the pristine DNA chromosomes that were present during infancy. Now science has progressed to where this process is better understood. It is possible that the body can repair loose ends of chromosomes, telomeres, through a metabolic enzyme process called *telomerase reverse transcriptase.*

While it could become painfully technical describing this process, let's just summarize by stating the fact that the body has processes for incorporating environmental information into DNA which allows a species to pass on acquired traits to its progeny; this is the basis of evolution. The system for encoding environmental responses into chromosomes is called RNA and uses *reverse transcriptase* as the enzymatic process to *transcribe* this additional information into the chromosome strands where they have the mission to replicate this acquired environment wisdom for the future benefit of the species.

When our self-generated energy is freed from pathogenesis, symptom relief, and excessive daily maintenance, then the next plateau upon which such restorative energy will manifest itself is on the sub-molecular level; the restoration then takes place *within* the cell. As these telomeres (chromosome strand ends) are repaired, when our cells go to replace themselves at least once every 11 months, they can become healthier during each regenerating cycle. The result of this process is *rejuvenation* wherein we witness ourselves getting younger with each passing season.

This is the miracle of a true Fountain of Youth and not a myth or a hoax. This is how Nature, in her will toward perfection, intended her handiwork to proceed. The key to this miraculous process functioning properly is that we simply *stop putting up obstacles* and allow this rejuvenating process to progress through its stages. This outcome ultimately requires more than merely adjusting our nutrition.

The 7 Principles of Optimal Health

With so many intrusions into your daily space, you don't want your already-too-complicated life further interrupted with complicated lifestyle modification strategies. The best programs of self-development follow simple rules that flow with the natural rhythm of your life.

A primary reason that people fail to meet their New Year's resolutions is that the new strategy is overly-complicated and thus becomes just another source of stress.

My book ***LIVING SUPERFOOD RESEARCH: Don't Get Sick, Stay Off Drugs and Live a Long Time*** introduced The Seven Principles of Optimal Health. These simple concepts crystalized after decades of detailed research on healthy living. I've shared these Seven Principles in presentations over many years, and audiences consistently welcome them. Let's use these principles as valuable tools to create space for perfect health as we reboot this month.

The **Seven Principles** which we intend to master as we deliberately create space for perfect health are:

1. **The Breath** - When it comes to prioritizing the most critical nutrients needed to survive, most people don't think of the primacy of breath awareness. Oxygen is the one nutrient that, when lacking, will cause the fastest injury and death. Mastery of breath awareness allows you to always be in control of the moment.

2. **Hydration** - Water makes up 70% of the surface of our planet. Similarly, your body is about 60 to 70% water, depending your level of healthy hydration. The brain is said to be 70% water and water is the greater percentage of our muscles, lungs and blood. We need water to regulate body temperature, move nutrients throughout the blood, transmit chemical communicators (hormones), remove waste, as well as to protect joints and organs.

3. **Food & Nutrition** - There are critical nutrients that we must regularly consume to be whole and healthy. The basics of food nutrition require us to consume vitamins, minerals, active enzymes, amino acids, protein, carbohydrates, essential fatty acids, and crude fiber, along with proper hydration, to provide the complete spectrum of daily nutrients needed for systemic function.

4. **Exercise** - For high quality living, the benefits we gain from exercise are crucial. Stress inhibits optimal functioning for most of our body systems. Hormones associated with

stress trigger hypertension, stroke, sleep disorders, indigestion, infertility, headaches, fatigue, muscle tension and chest pains, as well as depression and anxiety. To achieve perfect health, our program must include stress-reducing exercise.

5. **Fasting & Detoxification** - I've done seasonal detoxification fasts 4 times a year for over 15 years. I begin to fast on the first days of Spring, Summer, Autumn and Winter. There's an extensive list of foods, herbs and supplements that are excellent detoxing agents and supply multiple benefits. Because of constant exposure to environmental toxins all around, it is to our advantage that we detox as part of a regular routine.

6. **Sleep & Rest** - Many of us are driven by constant demands which include work, recreational activities, social media, electronic entertainment, and other commitments. As such, sleep is one area where we habitually sacrifice quality time to squeeze other in priorities. Sleep is just as important as the other six Principles and sleep deprivation is a major problem in society today.

7. **Psycho-Spiritual Orientation** – There's no debating the critical impact of mental and spiritual clarity on our health. The influence that the brain has over the body is powerful. We must comprehend how profoundly psychology and spirituality affect bodily function. We study these processes to gain every possible advantage to achieve vitality, longevity and disease-free living.

In the book Living Superfood Research these Seven Principles cover an extensive chapter. Each requires multiple pages of description of various approaches we can use. Living Superfood Research is the textbook used for the certification course during our annual retreat to Jamaica.

You work to attain mastery as you create space within your life for perfect health. I highly recommend that you get my Research book for more comprehensive instruction. I will guarantee that you will find it one of the most useful books on natural health in your library.

The option to live this way is available to nearly everyone who would so commit themselves. Unfortunately, there is immense negative reinforcement within the larger society to reject these types of self-transforming changes. It never fails to surprise one to hear the variety of excuses that people will drag out to continue living a restricted yet familiar existence. People stretch to rationalize as to why this lifestyle would be too inconvenient for them. What makes it even more paradoxical is that parents will unconsciously subject their children to a spectrum of compromises, unhealthy food and self-restriction. We claim we love our children yet don't take the time to properly research as to which factors will prove vital toward improving their chances to succeed within this society.

The challenge for those suffering advanced symptoms of chronic disease is that it's late in the game but still not too late. If we are still breathing, reasoning and can at least walk and engage in moderate physical activity, we have a chance to thrive. This miracle of rejuvenation begins with our Word — *Speaking-into-Being*. Isn't it amazing that certain words uttered with authenticity can trigger life-enhancing processes that will persist for many decades? Isn't it a miracle that we

79 | Chapter 7 — Four Stages of Healing

can Speak-into-Being for ourselves extended and enhanced longevity?

Once our self-generated energy has enabled us to rise to the perception and mastery of our True Divinity, then we can finally grasp the significance of what the **Uttered Word** is capable of.

I AM young again and I want each of you to stand up and reclaim your youthful vitality, resistance to disease, and longevity!

Four Stages of Healing
by Keidi Awadu / OFF-THE-WEIGHT

Eliminate the course of pathogenesis
1) Correct nutrient deficiencies
2) Eliminate environmental corrupters
3) Re-establish psycho-logical stability
4) Create homeostasis (healthy balance) throughout the body systems.

Rejuvenate on the cellular level
1) Every minute the body replaces 300 million of tens of trillions of cells
2) With aging DNA chromosome ends (telomeres) lose integrity & make incomplete copies
3) Through RNA our body repairs telomeres
4) New cells are stronger than those they replaced and the body's organs rejuvenate.

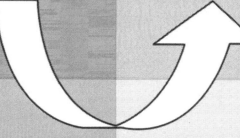

Remove the disease and symptoms
1) Reverse the internal disorder which causes disease
2) The disease loses its base & disappears
3) Symptoms which accompanied the disease are no longer needed
4) The body presents itself as healed of disease

Release energy that was misdirected
1) The body no longer wastes energy on battling disease and symptoms
2) During our sleep cycle more energy is avaiable to correct acute & chronic issues
3) The pace of nocturnal restoration speeds up
4) We awake refreshed, with more vital energy and feel more in control of our lives